CW0048699O

My Plant Based Everyday Diet

Easy & Tasteful Recipes
for your Diet

Joanna Vinson

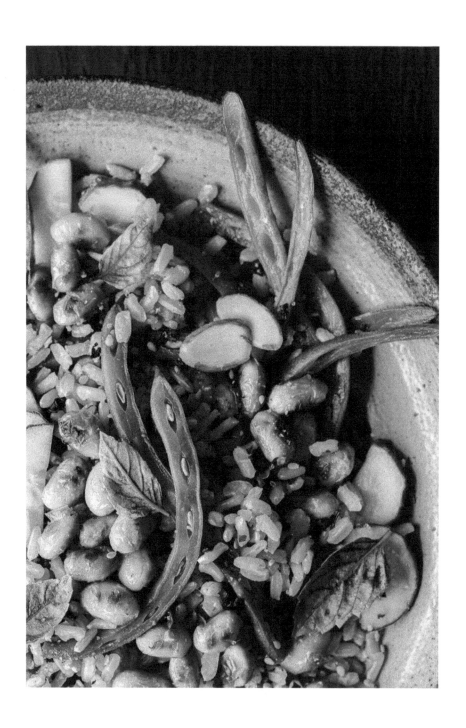

Table of Contents

Vegetable Lo Mein

Preparation Time: 10 minutes | Cooking Time: 15 minutes | Servings: 4

Ingredients:

- 8 ounces of spaghetti noodles

- 2 cups vegetable broth

- 1 teaspoon sesame oil

- 1 teaspoon ginger paste

- 1 teaspoon minced garlic

- 1 tablespoon soy sauce

- 1 tablespoon vinegar

- 1 teaspoon red chili paste

- 1 teaspoon brown sugar

- 1 teaspoon coconut oil

- ½ cup carrots, thinly sliced

- ½ cup cabbages, thinly sliced

- ½ cup broccoli florets

- salt and pepper to taste

- ½ cup green scallions

- Toasted sesame seeds for garnish

Directions:

- Place the spaghetti noodles and vegetable broth in the Pressure pot.

- Close the lid and set the vent to the Sealing position. Press the Pressure Cook or Manual button and adjust the cooking time to 8 minutes. Do quick pressure release and drain the noodles. Set the noodles aside to cool.

- Meanwhile, mix the sesame oil, ginger paste, garlic, soy sauce, vinegar, chili paste, and brown sugar. Set aside.

- Clean the inner pot and place it in the Pressure pot.

- Press the Sauté button and heat the oil. Sauté the carrots, cabbages, and broccoli florets. Season with salt and pepper to taste. Stir for 3 minutes.

- Add in the noodles and the sauce prepared earlier.

- Toss to coat the noodles and vegetables.

- Press the Cancel button to turn off the cooking.

- Garnish with scallions and sesame seeds before serving.

Nutrition:

Calories 120 | Total Fat 3g | Saturated Fat 1g | Total Carbs 20g | Net Carbs 16g | Protein 4g | Sugar: 3g | Fiber: 4g | Sodium: 75mg | Potassium: 155mg | Phosphorus: 74mg

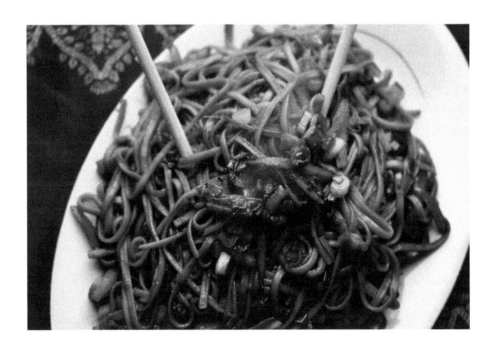

Herb and Vegetable Brown Rice

Preparation Time: 10 minutes | Cooking Time: 25 minutes | Servings: 6

Ingredients:

- 1 ½ tablespoon olive oil

- 1 cup onion, chopped

- 4 cloves of garlic, minced

- ½ cup red bell pepper, chopped

- ½ cup celery, chopped

- ¼ teaspoon dried oregano

- 1 ½ cup long-grain brown rice

- 1 ¾ cup water

- salt and pepper to taste

- ½ cup fresh parsley, minced

Directions:

• Press the Sauté button on the Pressure pot and heat the olive oil. Sauté the onion and garlic until fragrant. Stir in the bell pepper, celery, and oregano for 2 minutes until the celery has wilted.

• Stir in the brown rice, water, salt, and pepper. Stir everything to combine.

• Press the Rice button and cook using the pre-set cooking time. Do natural pressure release.

• Once the lid is open, fluff the rice and garnish with chopped parsley.

Nutrition:

• Calories 233 | Total Fat 6g | Saturated Fat 1g | Total Carbs 40g | Net Carbs 37g | Protein 6g | Sugar: 2g | Fiber: 3g | Sodium: 35mg | Potassium: 242mg | Phosphorus: 181mg

Kung Pao Brussels Sprouts

Preparation Time: 5 minutes | Cooking Time: 4 hours and 5 minutes | Servings: 4

Ingredients:

- 2 pounds Brussels sprouts, halved

- ½ cup of water

- 2 tablespoons extra-virgin olive oil

- salt and pepper to taste

- 1 tablespoon sesame oil

- 2 cloves of garlic, minced

- ½ cup of soy sauce

- 2 teaspoons apple cider vinegar

- 1 tablespoon hoisin sauce

- 1 tablespoon brown sugar

- 2 teaspoons garlic chili sauce

- 1 tablespoon cornstarch + 2 tablespoons water

- Sesame seeds for garnish

• Green onions for garnish

• 2 tablespoons chopped roasted peanuts

Directions:

• Place the Brussels sprouts and water in the Pressure pot and drizzle over the olive oil. Season with salt and pepper to taste. Close the lid but do not seal the vent.

• Press the Slow Cook button and adjust the cooking time to 4 hours.

• Take the broccoli out and set it aside.

• To the inner pot, stir in the sesame oil and press the Sauté button. Stir in the garlic for 30 seconds.

• Add in the water and bring to a boil.

• Stir in the soy sauce, apple cider vinegar, hoisin sauce, brown sugar, and garlic sauce. Bring to a boil and add in the cornstarch slurry until the sauce thickens.

• Add the slow-cooked broccoli into the sauce.

• Garnish with sesame seeds, green onions, and roasted peanuts before serving.

Nutrition:

Calories 343 | Total Fat 16g | Saturated Fat 3g | Total Carbs 43g | Net Carbs 32g | Protein 13g | Sugar: 20g | Fiber: 11g | Sodium: 757mg | Potassium: 1151mg | Phosphorus: 257mg

Parsnips and Carrots

Preparation Time: 5 minutes | Cooking Time: 10 minutes | Servings: 4

Ingredients:

- 1 tablespoon olive oil

- 2 cloves of garlic, minced

- 2 pounds carrots, peeled and sliced

- 2 pounds parsnips, peeled and sliced

- ½ cup of water

- ¼ cup maple syrup

- Salt and pepper to taste

- Fresh parsley, chopped

Directions:

- Press the Sauté button on the Pressure pot and heat the oil.

- Sauté the garlic for 30 seconds until fragrant. Stir in the carrots and parsnips for 3 minutes.

• Pour in water and maple syrup. Season with salt and pepper to taste.

• Close the lid and set the vent to the Sealing position.

• Press the Pressure Cooker or Manual button and adjust the cooking time to 6 minutes.

• Do natural pressure release.

• Once the lid is open, garnish with parsley.

Nutrition:

Calories 356 | Total Fat 5g | Saturated Fat 0.7g | Total Carbs 78g | Net Carbs 60g | Protein 6g | Sugar: 34g | Fiber: 18g | Sodium: 192mg | Potassium: 1745mg | Phosphorus: 257mg

Vegetarian Pad Thai

Preparation Time: 10 minutes | Cooking Time: 9 minutes | Servings: 4

Ingredients:

- ½ cup of soy sauce

- 1 tablespoon fresh lime juice

- 2 tablespoons of rice wine vinegar

- 3 tablespoons coconut aminos

- 1/3 cup granulated sugar

- 1 tablespoon vegetable oil

- 12 ounces extra-firm tofu, sliced

- 1 onion, chopped

- 1 clove garlic, minced

- 10 ounces Pad Thai rice noodles

- 2 cups vegetable stock

- 2 tablespoons shredded radish

- 1 cup bean sprouts

- 1 medium carrot, peeled and shredded

- ¼ cup unsalted peanuts, roasted

- 3 scallions, chopped

- 1 medium lime, cut into wedges

Directions:

- In a mixing bowl, combine the soy sauce, lime juice, wine vinegar, coconut aminos, and sugar. Set aside.

- Press the Sauté button on the Pressure pot and heat the olive. Brown the tofu for 3 minutes on each side. Set aside.

- Sauté the onion and garlic for 30 seconds until fragrant.

- Add the rice noodles, tofu, and vegetable stock. Close the lid and set the vent to the Sealing position.

- Press the Pressure Cooker or Manual button and adjust the cooking time to 6 minutes.

- Do quick pressure release. Once the lid is open, drain the noodles and set them aside.

- Place the noodles in bowls and top with radish, bean sprouts, carrots, peanuts, scallions, and lime wedges.

- Drizzle with the prepared sauce.

Nutrition:

Calories 559 | Total Fat 12g | Saturated Fat 4g | Total Carbs 93g | Net Carbs g | Protein 17g | Sugar: 23g | Fiber: 4g | Sodium: 432mg | Potassium: 521mg | Phosphorus: 125mg

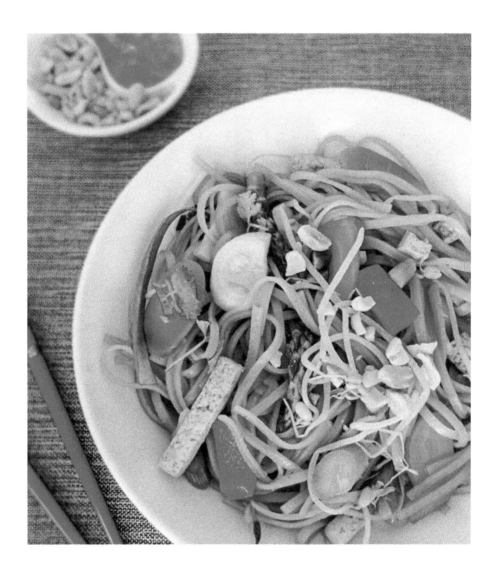

Red Curry Vegetables

Preparation Time: 5 minutes | Cooking Time: 15 minutes | Servings: 4

Ingredients:

- 1 onion, chopped

- 3 cloves garlic, minced

- 2 ½ cups chopped cauliflower florets

- 2 ½ cups cubed sweet potato

- 1 can coconut milk

- 1 can diced tomatoes

- 3 tablespoon red curry paste

- 2 teaspoons soy sauce

- 1 teaspoon turmeric

- 1 cup of water

- A bunch of kale leaves

- Fresh lime juice

- Fresh cilantro leaves

Directions:

• Place the onions and garlic in the Pressure pot. Add a teaspoon of water. Press the Sauté button and do water sauté for 1 minute.

• Stir in the cauliflower, sweet potato, milk, tomatoes, red curry paste, soy sauce, and turmeric. Add water.

• Close the lid and set the vent to the Sealing position.

• Press the Pressure Cooker or Manual button and adjust the cooking time to 10 minutes.

• Do quick pressure release.

• Once the lid is open, press the Sauté button and add the kale leaves. Cook for 3 more minutes until the kale leaves are wilted.

• Serve with lime juice and cilantro leaves.

Nutrition:

Calories 70 | Total Fat 1g | Saturated Fat 0g | Total Carbs 14g | Net Carbs 9g | Protein 3g | Sugar: 6g | Fiber:5 g | Sodium: 172mg | Potassium: 615mg | Phosphorus: 84mg

Vegetable Chow Mein

Preparation Time: 5 minutes | Cooking Time: 10 minutes | Servings: 5

Ingredients:

- 4 cups vegetable broth

- 2 tablespoon dark soy sauce

- 1 teaspoon sesame oil

- 1 tablespoon vinegar

- 1 tablespoons sriracha sauce

- 1 tablespoon brown sugar

- 16 ounces Hakka noodles

- 1 teaspoon grated ginger

- 1 teaspoon grated garlic

- 1 cup cabbage, thinly sliced

- ½ cup celery, chopped

- 2 carrots, peeled and julienned

- 1 cup snow peas, trimmed

- 1 cup broccoli florets

- ½ cup green onion, chopped

Directions:

- In a bowl, mix the vegetable broth, soy sauce, sesame oil, sriracha sauce, and brown sugar. Whisk and set aside.

- Press the Sauté button on the Pressure pot and pour the prepared sauce. Spread the noodles over the sauce. Top with grated ginger, garlic, cabbage, celery, and carrots.

- Close the lid and set the vent to the Sealing position.

- Press the Pressure Cooker or Manual button. Adjust the cooking time to 5 minutes.

- Do quick pressure release.

- Once the lid is open, press the Sauté button and stir in the snow peas and broccoli. Cook for 5 minutes.

- Garnish with green onion.

Nutrition:

Calories 172 | Total Fat 2g | Saturated Fat 0.4g | Total Carbs 33g | Net Carbs 31g | Protein 5g | Sugar: 5g | Fiber: 2g | Sodium: 295mg | Potassium: 201mg | Phosphorus: 56mg

Pressure pot Carrots

Preparation Time: 5 minutes | Cooking Time: 8 minutes | Servings: 4

Ingredients:

• 2 pounds fresh carrots, cut into thick strips

• 1 cup of water

• 1 tablespoon olive oil

• 1 teaspoon fresh thyme

Directions:

• Place the carrots and water in the Pressure pot.

• Lock the lid and set the vent to the Sealing position.

• Press the Pressure Cooker or Manual button and adjust the cooking time to 5 minutes.

• Once the timer sets off, do a quick pressure release and drain the carrots.

• Clean the inner pot.

• Press the Sauté button and heat the oil. Stir in the thyme to toast and add in the carrots. Stir fry for 3 minutes.

Nutrition:

Calories 109 | Total Fat 4g | Saturated Fat 0.5g | Total Carbs 19g | Net Carbs 12g | Protein 2g | Sugar: 8g | Fiber: 7g | Sodium: 132mg | Potassium: 534mg | Phosphorus: 68mg

Pressure pot Carrot Soup

Preparation Time: 10 minutes | Cooking Time: 20 minutes | Servings: 4

Ingredients:

- 1 tablespoon olive oil

- 1 onion, chopped

- 4 cloves garlic, minced

- 1 carrot, peeled and diced

- 1 teaspoon dried oregano

- ½ teaspoon paprika

- ½ teaspoon cumin

- ½ teaspoon chopped mint

- ½ cup coarse bulgur

- salt and pepper to taste

- 4 cups vegetable stock

- 2 cups baby spinach

- 1 lemon juice, freshly squeezed

Directions:

• Press the Sauté button on the Pressure pot and heat the oil.

• Sauté the onion and garlic for 30 seconds or until fragrant.

• Stir in the carrot, oregano, paprika, cumin, mint, bulgur, and vegetable stock. Season with salt and pepper to taste.

• Close the lid and set the vent to the Sealing position.

• Press the Pressure Cook or Manual button and adjust the cooking time to 15 minutes.

• Do quick pressure release.

• Once the lid is open, press the Sauté button and stir in the spinach. Cook for 3 minutes or until the spinach has wilted.

• Drizzle with lemon juice before serving.

Nutrition:

Calories 118 | Total Fat 6g | Saturated Fat g | Total Carbs 11g | Net Carbs g | Protein 7g | Sugar: 2g | Fiber: 2.5g | Sodium: 33mg | Potassium: 273mg | Phosphorus:79 mg

Summer Vegetable Soup

Preparation Time: 10 minutes | Cooking Time: 20 minutes | Servings: 4

Ingredients:

- 4 cups vegetable broth

- 1 14-ounce can diced tomatoes

- 2 tablespoon tomato paste

- 1 small yellow onion, diced

- 1 red bell pepper, diced

- 1 small zucchini, chopped

- 2 ears of corn, shucked

- 1 tablespoon fresh lemon juice

- 1 tablespoon fresh parsley, chopped

- salt and pepper to taste

Directions:

- Place all ingredients in the Pressure pot and give a good stir.

• Press the Broth/Soup button and adjust the cooking time to 20 minutes. Cook on high pressure.

• Do quick pressure release.

Nutrition:

Calories 97 | Total Fat 1g | Saturated Fat 0.2g | Total Carbs 22g | Net Carbs 17g | Protein 4g | Sugar: 7g | Fiber: 5g | Sodium: 132mg | Potassium: 547mg | Phosphorus: 100mg

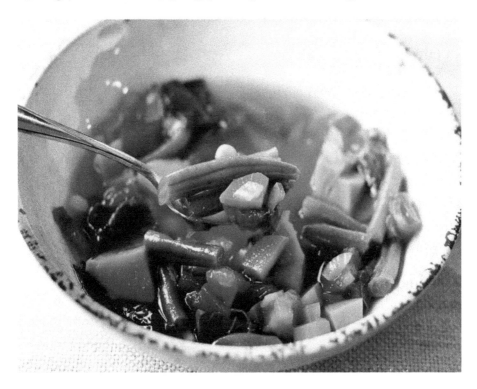

Hibachi Mushroom Steak

Preparation Time: minutes | Cooking Time: minutes | Servings: 2

Ingredients:

- 1/3 cup soy sauce

- 2 tablespoons white vinegar

- 1 tablespoon grated ginger

- 1 tablespoon minced garlic

- pound large chestnut mushrooms stems removed

- 1 zucchini, sliced in rounds

- 1 yellow onion.

- 1 tablespoon granulated sugar

- Salt and pepper to taste

Directions:

- Place all ingredients in a bowl and allow ingredients to marinate in the fridge for at least 30 minutes.

• Pour in the Pressure pot all ingredients.

• Close the lid and set the vent to the Sealing position.

• Press the Pressure Cook or Manual button and cook on high. Adjust the cooking time to 5 minutes.

• Do natural pressure release.

Nutrition:

Calories 208 | Total Fat 8g | Saturated Fat 2g | Total Carbs 26g | Net Carbs 22g | Protein 11g | Sugar: 18g | Fiber: 4g | Sodium: 650mg | Potassium: 950mg | Phosphorus: 265mg

Lemony Rice and Vegetable Soup

Preparation Time: 10 minutes | Cooking Time: 20 minutes | Servings: 4

Ingredients:

- 1 tablespoon extra-virgin olive oil

- 1 yellow onion, chopped

- 2 cloves of garlic, minced

- 2 large carrots, diced

- 2 stalks celery, diced

- ½ large fennel bulb, diced

- ½ teaspoon ground cumin

- 1 cup brown basmati rice

- 2 handful spinach

- 6 cups vegetable broth

- salt and pepper to taste

- 4 tablespoons fresh lemon juice

Directions:

• Press the Sauté button on the Pressure pot and heat the oil.

• Sauté the onion and garlic for 30 seconds until fragrant.

• Stir in the carrots, celery, fennel, and cumin. Stir for 2 minutes until the vegetables are wilted.

• Add in the rice, spinach, and broth. Season with salt and pepper to taste.

• Stir the ingredients until well-combined.

• Close the lid and set the vent to the Sealing position.

• Press the Rice button and cook using the preset cooking time.

• Do natural pressure release.

• Once the lid is open, drizzle with lemon juice then fluff the rice.

Nutrition:

Calories 245 | Total Fat 5g | Saturated Fat 0.8g | Total Carbs 45g | Net Carbs 41g | Protein 5g | Sugar: 5g | Fiber: 4g | Sodium: 84mg | Potassium: 418mg | Phosphorus: 196mg

Vegetable Pho Soup

Preparation Time: 10 minutes | Cooking Time: 40 minutes | Servings: 4

Ingredients:

- 2 tablespoons olive oil

- 1 onion, quartered

- 5 whole star anise pods

- 1 tablespoon fennel seeds

- 1 tablespoon coriander seeds

- 1 cinnamon stick

- ½ tablespoon whole black peppercorns

- 1 cup dried mushrooms

- 1 1-inch ginger, peeled

- 2 kaffir lime leaves

- 2 bay leaves

- 2 celery stalks, chopped roughly

- 1 large carrot, chopped roughly

- 4 cups of water

- salt to taste

- 2 cup broccoli florets

- 2 tablespoons cilantro, chopped

- 1 cup straw mushrooms

- 8 ounces shiitake mushrooms

- 1 small zucchini, chopped

- 1 cup mung bean sprouts

- 1 cup basil leaves

- 1 lime, cut into wedges

- Sriracha sauce

Directions:

- Press the Sauté button and heat the oil. Toast the onion, anise, fennel seeds, coriander, cinnamon stick, black peppercorns, dried mushrooms, ginger, kaffir lime leaves, and bay leaves. Stir for 2 minutes until fragrant.

- Add in the celery and carrots and stir for another 3 minutes before pouring in water. Season with salt to taste.

- Close the lid and set the vent to the Sealing position.

• Press the Broth/Soup button and cook using the preset cooking time. Do quick pressure release once the timer has set off.

• Once the lid is open, remove the solids. Add in the broccoli, cilantro, mushrooms, and zucchini.

• Close the lid again and set the vent to the Sealing position. Press the Pressure Cook or Manual button and adjust the cooking time to 5 minutes.

• Do natural pressure release.

• Garnish with bean sprouts, basil leaves, and lime wedges before serving. Drizzle with sriracha sauce if desired.

Nutrition:

Calories 171 | Total Fat 9g | Saturated Fat 1g | Total Carbs 23g | Net Carbs 17g | Protein 6g | Sugar: 6g | Fiber: 6g | Sodium: 215mg | Potassium: 511mg | Phosphorus: 143mg

Veggie Macaroni

Preparation Time: 10 minutes | Cooking Time: 20 minutes | Servings: 4

Ingredients:

- 2 cups dry macaroni

- 2 cups of water

- 1 ½ cups marinara sauce

- ½ cup of coconut milk

- 1 cup frozen veggies of your choice

- 2 tablespoons nutritional yeast

- salt and pepper to taste

Directions:

- Add all ingredients to the Pressure pot and give a good stir.

- Close the lid and set the vent to the Sealing position.

- Press the Multigrain button and cook on high. Adjust the cooking time to 20 minutes.

• Do natural pressure release.

Nutrition:

Calories 330 | Total Fat 9g | Saturated Fat 7g | Total Carbs 51g | Net Carbs 56g | Protein 11g | Sugar: 8g | Fiber: 5g | Sodium: 306mg | Potassium: 692mg | Phosphorus: 171mg

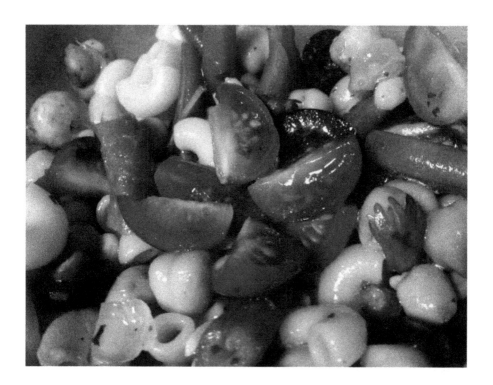

Pressure pot Broccoli

Preparation Time: 10 minutes | Cooking Time: 10 minutes | Servings: 4

Ingredients:

• 2 heads broccoli, cut into florets

• 2 tablespoons coconut oil

• salt and pepper to taste

• 3 tablespoons nutritional yeast

Directions:

• Pour a cup of water into the Pressure pot and place a steamer basket or trivet.

• Place the broccoli florets in the steamer basket.

• Close the lid and set the vent to the Sealing position.

• Press the Steam button and cook for 10 minutes.

• Do quick pressure release.

• Once the lid is open, take the broccoli out and place it in a bowl.

• Drizzle with oil and season with salt, pepper, and nutritional yeast.

• Toss to combine everything.

Nutrition:

Calories 88 | Total Fat 7g | Saturated Fat 4g | Total Carbs 3g | Net Carbs 2g | Protein 4g | Sugar: 0.3g | Fiber: 1g | Sodium: 406mg | Potassium: 323mg | Phosphorus: 29mg

Vegan Jambalaya

Preparation Time: 10 minutes | Cooking Time: 25 minutes | Servings: 4

Ingredients:

- 1 tablespoon oil

- 1 onion, diced

- 1 green bell pepper, seeded and diced

- 3 ribs of celery, diced

- 4 cloves of garlic, minced

- 1 ½ cup long-grain white rice

- 1 can small diced tomatoes

- 1 tablespoon Cajun seasoning

- 2 teaspoons smoked paprika

- 3 cups vegetable broth

- ¼ cup chopped parsley

- salt and pepper to taste

Directions:

• Press the Sauté button on the Pressure pot and heat the oil.

• Sauté the onion, green bell pepper, celery, and garlic. Stir for 2 minutes until fragrant.

• Add in the rest of the ingredients and give a good stir.

• Close the lid and set the vent to the Sealing position.

• Press the Rice button and cook on low pressure.

• Do natural pressure release.

Nutrition:

Calories 319 | Total Fat 4g | Saturated Fat 0.7g | Total Carbs 63g | Net Carbs 60g | Protein 6g | Sugar: 3g | Fiber: 3g | Sodium: 165mg | Potassium: 293mg | Phosphorus: 109mg

Pressure pot Veggie Curry

Preparation Time: 5 minutes | Cooking Time: 10 minutes | Servings: 4

Ingredients:

- 1 tablespoon coconut oil

- 1 onion, diced

- 1 teaspoon mustard seeds

- 4 cloves of garlic, minced

- 2 tablespoons Indian curry powder

- 1 teaspoon grated ginger

- 1 cup vegetable broth

- 1 cup light coconut milk

- 1 butternut squash, seeded and diced

- 1 red bell pepper, diced

- 1 14-ounce canned chickpeas, drained and rinsed

- 2 tablespoons brown sugar

- ½ teaspoon salt

• Chopped cilantro for garnish

Directions:

• Set the Pressure pot to the Sauté mode and add oil. Stir in the onion, mustard seeds, garlic, curry powder, and ginger. Keep stirring for 1 minute until fragrant.

• Add in the broth, coconut milk, squash, bell pepper, and chickpeas. Season with brown sugar and salt.

• Close the lid and set the vent to the Sealing position.

• Press the Pressure Cook or Manual button and cook on high. Adjust the cooking time to 10 minutes.

• Do quick pressure release.

• Garnish with cilantro before serving.

Nutrition:

Calories 353 | Total Fat 21g | Saturated Fat 16g | Total Carbs 37g | Net Carbs 27g | Protein 10g | Sugar: 11g | Fiber: 10g | Sodium: 397mg | Potassium: 515mg | Phosphorus: 173mg

Potato Curry

Preparation Time: 10 minutes | Cooking Time: 30 minutes | Servings: 5

Ingredients:

- 1 teaspoon oil

- 1 yellow onion, chopped

- 4 cloves of garlic, minced

- 5 cups baby potatoes, scrubbed clean

- 2 tablespoons curry powder

- 2 cups of water

- 1 can coconut milk, full fat

- Salt and pepper to taste

- 1 teaspoon chili pepper flakes

- 2 cups green beans, chopped into inch-thick pieces

- 3 tablespoons arrowroot powder + 4 tablespoons water

Directions:

• Set the Sauté button on the Pressure pot and heat oil. Sauté the onion and garlic for 30 seconds until fragrant.

• Stir in the potatoes and curry powder. Keep stirring for 3 minutes.

• Add water and coconut milk. Season with salt, pepper, and chili flakes.

• Close the lid and set the vent to the Sealing position.

• Press the Pressure Cook or Manual button and cook on high. Adjust the cooking time to 20 minutes.

• Do quick pressure release.

• Once the lid is open, press the Sauté button and add in the green beans. Cook for 5 minutes.

• Stir in the arrowroot slurry and allow to thicken for 5 more minutes.

Nutrition:

Calories 187 | Total Fat 4g | Saturated Fat 0.6g | Total Carbs 36g | Net Carbs 29g | Protein 5g | Sugar: 6g | Fiber: 7g | Sodium: 61mg | Potassium: 917mg | Phosphorus: 133mg

Vegan Tofu and Little Potato Stew

Preparation Time: 10 minutes | Cooking Time: 28 minutes | Servings: 5

Ingredients:

- 2 tablespoons olive oil

- 1 block (350g) extra-firm tofu, cubed

- ½ cup chopped yellow onion

- 2 cloves of garlic

- 1 ½ cups carrots

- 1 ½ cup chopped celery

- 1 ½ pounds baby potatoes, scrubbed

- 1 cup frozen peas

- 2 tablespoons soy sauce

- 6 cups vegetable broth

- 3 tablespoons tomato paste

- 1 cup of water

- salt and pepper to taste

- 2 tablespoons cornstarch + 3 tablespoons water

Directions:

- Press the Sauté button on the Pressure pot and heat the oil.

- Sear the tofu on all sides until lightly golden.

- Stir in the onion and garlic until fragrant.

- Add the carrots, celery, potatoes, and peas. Stir-fry the vegetables for 2 minutes.

- Pour in the water and season with soy sauce, salt, and pepper. Add the tomato paste.

- Close the lid and set the vent to the Sealing position.

- Press the Meat/Stew button and adjust the cooking time to 20 minutes.

- Do quick pressure release.

- Once the lid is open, press the Sauté button and stir in the cornstarch slurry and cook for 5

minutes until the sauce thickens.

Nutrition:

Calories 152 | Total Fat 7g | Saturated Fat 2g | Total Carbs 17g | Net Carbs 14g | Protein 6g | Sugar: 3g | Fiber: 3g | Sodium: 880mg | Potassium: 975mg | Phosphorus: 436mg

Pressure pot Cabbage

Preparation Time: 10 minutes | Cooking Time: 9vminutes | Servings: 6

Ingredients:

- 1 onion, diced

- 2 cups vegetable broth

- 1 teaspoon oregano

- ½ teaspoon thyme

- 1 head of green cabbage, chopped

- salt and pepper to taste

Directions:

• Press the Sauté button on the Pressure pot and cook the onion with a tablespoon of vegetable broth for 3 minutes. Stir in the oregano and thyme and cook for another minute.

• Stir in the remaining broth and cabbages. Season with salt and pepper to taste.

• Close the lid and set the vent to the Sealing position.

• Press the Pressure Cook or Manual button and cook on high. Adjust the cooking time to 5 minutes.

• Do natural pressure release.

Nutrition:

Calories 69 | Total Fat 3g | Saturated Fat 0.5g | Total Carbs 11g | Net Carbs 8g | Protein 2g | Sugar: 5g | Fiber: 3g | Sodium: 416mg | Potassium: 340mg | Phosphorus: 57mg

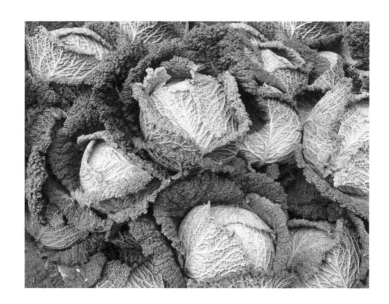

Pressure pot Homestyle Veggies

Preparation Time: 5 minutes | Cooking Time: 20 minutes | Servings: 4

Ingredients:

- 1 cup vegetable broth

- ½ pound whole carrots, peeled and roughly chopped

- pound fresh green beans, trimmed

- 1 ½ pounds red potatoes, cut in half

- salt and pepper to taste

Directions:

- Pour broth into the Pressure pot.

- Place the vegetables on a steamer basket or trivet and season with salt and pepper to taste.

- Close the lid and set the vent to the Sealing position.

- Press the Steam button and cook using the pre-set cooking time.

- Do natural pressure release.

Nutrition:

Calories 122 | Total Fat 0g | Saturated Fat 0g | Total Carbs 26g | Net Carbs g | Protein 4g | Sugar: 4g | Fiber: 4g | Sodium: 39mg | Potassium: 673mg | Phosphorus: 235mg

Pressure pot Steamed Vegetables

Preparation Time: 10 minutes | Cooking Time: 5 minutes | Servings: 6

Ingredients:

- 1 cup of water

- 2 cups raw baby carrots

- 2 cups raw cauliflower florets

- 2 cups raw broccoli florets

Directions:

- Pour water into the Pressure pot and place a steamer basket or trivet inside.

- Place the vegetables in the steamer basket.

- Close the lid and set the vent to the Sealing position.

- Press the Steam button and cook using the pre-set cooking time.

- Do natural pressure release.

Nutrition:

Calories 27 | Total Fat 0.3g | Saturated Fat 0g | Total Carbs 6g | Net Carbs 4g | Protein 2g | Sugar: 2g | Fiber:2 g | Sodium: 40mg | Potassium: 250mg | Phosphorus: 38mg

Pressure pot Vegetable Korma

Preparation Time: 10 minutes | Cooking Time: 27minutes | Servings: 4

Ingredients:

- 1 large sweet onion, chopped

- 15 raw cashews, soaked in water overnight

- 1 1-inch ginger, sliced

- 4 cloves garlic, peeled

- 2 tablespoons coconut oil

- 6 whole black peppercorns

- 4 green cardamoms

- 4 whole cloves

- 1 bay leaf

- ½ cup tomato puree

- 2 tablespoons garam masala or curry powder

- ½ teaspoon sugar

- 1 large potato, peeled and diced

- 2 medium carrots, peeled and diced

- ¼ cup of frozen green peas

- 1 cup of coconut milk

- ½ cup of water

- Juice from half of lemon

- salt and pepper to taste

- 2 tablespoons chopped cilantro

Directions:

- Place the onion, cashews, ginger, and garlic in a blender and pulse until smooth. Set aside.

- Press the Sauté button on the Pressure pot and heat the oil. Toast the peppercorns, cardamoms, cloves, bay leaf for 2 minutes until fragrant.

- Stir in the onion-cashew paste and stir for 3 minutes. Add the tomato puree and stir to remove the brown bits at the bottom.

- Add the garam masala and sugar. Stir in the vegetables. Continue stirring for 2 minutes.

- Stir in the coconut milk, water, and lemon juice. Season with salt and pepper to taste.

• Press the Cancel button and close the lid. Set the vent to the Sealing position.

• Press the Meat/Stew button and cook on the lowest pre-set cooking button.

• Do natural pressure release.

• Serve with chopped cilantro.

Nutrition:

Calories 189 | Total Fat 21g | Saturated Fat 11g | Total Carbs 14g | Net Carbs 11g | Protein 4g | Sugar: 4g | Fiber: 3g | Sodium: 341mg | Potassium: 509mg | Phosphorus: 236mg

One-Pot Vegetarian Linguine

Preparation Time: 10 minutes | Cooking Time: 10 minutes | Servings: 6

Ingredients:

- 1 tablespoon olive oil

- 2 small onions, chopped

- 1 clove garlic, minced

- ½ pound fresh cremini mushrooms, sliced

- 1 large tomato, chopped

- 2 medium zucchinis, thinly sliced

- 4 tablespoons nutritional yeast

- salt and pepper

- 6 ounces uncooked linguine

- 3 cups of water

- 2 tablespoons cornstarch + 3 tablespoons water

Directions:

• Press the Sauté button on the Pressure pot. Heat the oil and sauté the onions and garlic for 1 minute until fragrant.

• Stir in the mushrooms and tomato. Stir for a minute.

• Add in the zucchini and season with nutritional yeast, salt, and pepper to taste.

• Add the linguine and water. Stir to combine.

• Close the lid and set the vent to the Sealing position.

• Press the Pressure Cook or Manual button and cook on high. Adjust the cooking time to 6 minutes.

• Do quick pressure release once the timer sets off.

• Open the lid and press the Sauté button. Stir in the cornstarch slurry and continue to stir until the sauce thickens.

Nutrition:

Calories 239 | Total Fat 3g | Saturated Fat 0.4g | Total Carbs 52g | Net Carbs 44g | Protein 8g | Sugar: 18g | Fiber:8 g | Sodium: 366mg | Potassium: 1286mg | Phosphorus: 162mg

Creamy Cauliflower and Broccoli Medley

Preparation Time: 5 minutes | Cooking Time: 5 minutes | Servings: 8

Ingredients:

- 2 pounds bag of cauliflower and broccoli florets mix

- 1 can coconut milk

- Zest of 1 lemon

- Juice from ½ lemon

- ¼ teaspoon garlic powder

- ¼ teaspoon oregano

- ¼ teaspoon dried parsley

- ¼ teaspoon dried basil

- 1/8 teaspoon onion powder

- salt and pepper to taste

Directions:

• Place all ingredients in the Pressure pot.

• Stir to combine everything.

• Close the lid and set the vent to the Sealing position.

• Press the Pressure Cooker or Manual button and cook on high. Adjust the cooking time to 5 minutes.

• Do natural pressure release.

Nutrition:

Calories 32 | Total Fat 0.6g | Saturated Fat 0g | Total Carbs 5g | Net Carbs 2g | Protein 4g | Sugar: 1g | Fiber:3 g | Sodium: 65mg | Potassium: 299mg | Phosphorus: 89mg

Potato and Carrot Medley

Preparation Time: 10 minutes | Cooking Time: 19 minutes | Servings: 6

Ingredients:

- 2 tablespoons extra virgin olive oil

- 1 onion, chopped

- 3 cloves of garlic, minced

- 4 pounds Yukon potatoes, cut into chunks

- 2 pounds carrots, sliced

- 1 teaspoon Italian seasoning mix

- salt and pepper to taste

- 1 ½ cup vegetable broth

- Fresh parsley for garnish

Directions:

- Press the Sauté button on the Pressure pot and heat the oil.

- Sauté the onion and garlic. Stir for 30 seconds until fragrant.

• Stir in the potatoes and carrots. Season with salt, pepper, and Italian seasoning mix. Stir for 3 minutes.

• Add in the broth.

• Close the lid and set the vent to the Sealing position.

• Press the Pressure Cooker or Manual button and cook on high. Adjust the cooking time to 15 minutes.

• Do natural pressure release.

• Once the lid is open, garnish with parsley before serving.

Nutrition:

Calories 341 | Total Fat 4g | Saturated Fat 0.8g | Total Carbs 71g | Net Carbs 60g | Protein 9g | Sugar: 11g | Fiber: 11g | Sodium: 354mg | Potassium: 1810mg | Phosphorus: 242mg

Pressure pot Vegetable Spaghetti

Preparation Time: 5 minutes | Cooking Time: 6 minutes | Servings: 6

Ingredients:

- 1 tablespoon olive oil

- 2 cloves of garlic, minced

- 4 ounces mushrooms, diced

- 1 large carrot, chopped

- 2 zucchinis, chopped

- 1 green bell pepper, diced

- ½ cup chopped basil

- 2 cups of water

- 8 ounces of spaghetti noodles

- 24 ounces pasta sauce

- salt and pepper to taste

Directions:

• Press the Sauté button on the Pressure pot.

• Heat the oil and stir in the garlic once the oil is hot. Add in the mushrooms and sauté for 4 minutes.

• Add the carrots, zucchini, and bell pepper. Stir for another 3 minutes. Add the basil.

• Deglaze the pot with water to remove the browned bits.

• Break the spaghetti pasta into the Pressure pot. Pour over the remaining water and pasta sauce. Season with salt and pepper to taste.

• Close the lid and set the vent to the Sealing position.

• Press the Pressure Cooker or Manual button and cook on high for 6 minutes.

• Do quick pressure release.

• Once the lid is open, give the pasta a good mix to combine everything.

Nutrition:

Calories 114 | Total Fat 3g | Saturated Fat 0.4g | Total Carbs 21g, Net Carbs 16g | Protein 5g | Sugar: 6g | Fiber: 5g | Sodium: 812mg | Potassium: 491mg | Phosphorus: 102mg

Lemon Couscous

Preparation Time: 10 minutes | Cooking Time: 24 minutes | Servings: 4

Ingredients:

- 1 cup pearl couscous
- 1 ¼ cup water
- 1 tablespoon olive oil
- ¾ cup sliced scallions
- 1 clove garlic, minced
- ¾ teaspoon salt
- ¼ teaspoon pepper
- 1 teaspoon lemon zest

Directions:

- Place couscous and water in the Pressure pot.
- Close the lid and set the vent to the Sealing position. Press the Rice button and cook using the preset cooking time.

• Once the timer sets off, open the lid and fluff the couscous. Remove from the Pressure pot and clean the inner pot.

• Return the inner pot into the Pressure pot and press the Sauté button. Heat the oil and sauté the scallions and garlic for 30 seconds until fragrant.

• Stir in the couscous and season with salt, pepper, and lemon zest.

• Stir for 3 minutes.

• Serve warm.

Nutrition:

Calories 81 | Total Fat 3g | Saturated Fat g0.5 | Total Carbs 11g | Net Carbs 10g | Protein 2g | Sugar: 0.5g | Fiber: 1g | Sodium: 5mg | Potassium: 79mg | Phosphorus: 17mg

Veggie Pasta Shells

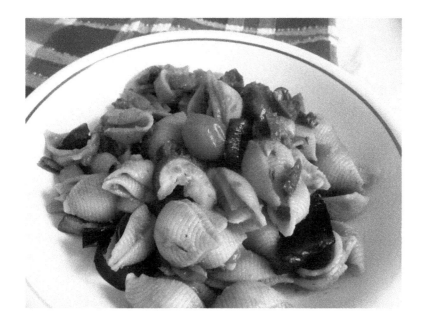

Preparation Time: 10 minutes | Cooking Time: 10 minutes | Servings: 6

Ingredients:

- 2 tablespoons olive oil

- 1 small onion, chopped

- 1 clove garlic, minced

- ½ bunch broccoli, cut into florets

- 1 cup shredded carrot

- ¼ cup basil leaves

- ½ cup marinara sauce

- 1 box pasta shells

- 4 tablespoons nutritional yeast

- salt and pepper to taste

Directions:

- Press the Sauté button on the Pressure pot and heat the oil.

- Sauté the onion and garlic until fragrant. Stir in the rest of the ingredients.

- Give a stir to combine.

- Close the lid and set the vent to the Sealing position.

- Press the Pressure Cook or Manual button and cook on high. Adjust the cooking time to 8 minutes.

- Once the timer sets off, do a quick pressure release.

Nutrition:

Calories 98 | Total Fat 5g | Saturated Fat 0.7g | Total Carbs 8g | Net Carbs 5g | Protein 5g | Sugar: 3g | Fiber: 3g | Sodium: 396mg | Potassium: 523mg | Phosphorus: 60mg

Veggies with Herbed Mushrooms

Preparation Time: 5 minutes | Cooking Time: 8 minutes | Servings: 6

Ingredients:

- 1 tablespoon coconut oil

- 1 onion, chopped

- 4 cloves garlic, minced

- 3 ounces shiitake mushrooms, sliced

- 3 ounces cremini mushrooms, sliced

- 3 ounces button mushrooms, sliced

- 1 teaspoon dried thyme

- 1 teaspoon Italian oregano

- salt and pepper to taste

- 12 ounces of frozen vegetables

- 1 cup vegetable broth

Directions:

• Press the Sauté button on the Pressure pot and heat the oil. Sauté the onion and garlic for 30 seconds until fragrant.

• Stir in the mushrooms and season with thyme, oregano, salt, and pepper. Stir for 2 minutes.

• Add in the rest of the ingredients.

• Close the lid and set the vent to the Sealing position.

• Press the Pressure Cook or Manual button and cook on high. Set the cooking time to 5 minutes.

• Do natural pressure release once the timer sets off.

Nutrition:

Calories 159 | Total Fat 3g | Saturated Fat 2g | Total Carbs 33g | Net Carbs 26g | Protein 5g | Sugar: 4g | Fiber: 7g | Sodium: 25mg | Potassium: 585mg | Phosphorus: 125mg

Simple Steamed Butternut Squash

Preparation Time: 10 minutes | Cooking Time: 10minutes | Servings: 4

Ingredients:

- 1 cup of water

- 1 medium butternut squash, peeled and sliced thickly

- 2 tablespoons extra virgin olive oil

- 1 tablespoon vegetable bouillon, cracked into powder

- salt and pepper to taste

Directions:

• Place a cup of water in the Pressure pot and place a trivet or steamer basket inside.

• In a bowl, season the butternut squash with olive oil, vegetable bouillon, salt, and pepper.

• Place in a heat-proof dish that will fit inside the Pressure pot.

• Place inside the Pressure pot and close the lid. Set the vent to the Sealing position.

• Press the Steam button and cook on high for 10 minutes.

• Do natural pressure release.

Nutrition:

Calories 57 | Total Fat 6g | Saturated Fat 3g | Total Carbs 1g | Net Carbs 0.5g | Protein 0.01g | Sugar: 0.005g | Fiber: 0.5g | Sodium: 60mg | Potassium: 9mg | Phosphorus:2 mg

Summer Squash and Mint Pasta

Preparation Time: 10 minutes | Cooking Time: 10 minutes | Servings: 5

Ingredients:

- 2 tablespoons olive oil

- 1 shallot, minced

- 1 cup sliced squash

- 1/3 cup mint, chopped

- 1 tablespoon lemon juice

- 12 ounces rigatoni pasta

- 4 tablespoons nutritional yeast

- salt and pepper to taste

- 1 ½ cups water

Directions:

- Press the Sauté button on the Pressure pot. Heat the oil.

• Sauté the shallots until fragrant. Add in the squash, mint, and the rest of the ingredients.

• Give a good stir.

• Close the lid and set the vent to the Sealing position.

• Press the Pressure Cook or Manual button. Adjust the cooking time to 7 minutes.

• Do natural pressure release.

Nutrition:

Calories 183 | Total Fat 7g | Saturated Fat 1g | Total Carbs 22g | Net Carbs 18g | Protein 8g | Sugar: 0.3g | Fiber: 4g | Sodium: 432mg | Potassium: 364mg | Phosphorus: 90mg

Root Vegetable and Squash Stew

Preparation Time: 5 minutes | Cooking Time: 25 minutes | Servings: 5

Ingredients:

- 1 tablespoon olive oil

- 1 red onion

- ½ small celeriac, sliced

- ½ butternut squash, seeded and sliced into chunks

- 1 sweet potato, peeled and cubed

- 2 carrots, peeled and cubed

- 1 teaspoon red wine vinegar

- 1 teaspoon dried thyme

- 1 bay leaf

- 1 tablespoon tomato puree

- 1 cup plum tomatoes, chopped

- salt and pepper to taste

- 1 tablespoon plain flour + 2 tablespoons cold water

Directions:

• Press the Sauté button on the Pressure pot and heat the oil. Sauté the onion and celeriac. Stir for 3 minutes.

• Add in the squash, sweet potato, and carrots. Stir for another minute.

• Stir in the red wine vinegar, thyme, bay leaf, tomato puree, and tomatoes. Season with salt and pepper to taste. Add a cup of water.

• Close the lid and set the vent to the Sealing position.

• Press the Meat/Stew button and adjust the cooking time to 20 minutes.

• Do quick pressure release.

• Once the lid is open, press the Sauté button and stir in the flour slurry. Cook for another 3 minutes until the sauce thickens.

Nutrition:

Calories 122 | Total Fat 3g | Saturated Fat 1g | Total Carbs 24g | Net Carbs 21g | Protein 1g | Sugar: 15g | Fiber: 3g | Sodium: 53mg | Potassium: 323mg | Phosphorus: 55mg

Veggie Tofu Pressure pot Stir Fry

Preparation Time: 5 minutes | Cooking Time: 15 minutes | Servings: 4

Ingredients:

- 3 tablespoons olive oil

- 1 block firm tofu, sliced

- 2 cloves garlic, minced

- 1 1-inch ginger, sliced thinly

- 2 fresh red chilis, chopped

- ½ head broccoli, cut into florets

- 4 baby corn, sliced

- 2 tablespoons soy sauce

- black pepper to taste

- ½ cup of water

- 1 tablespoon cornstarch + 2 tablespoons water

- 3 tablespoons sesame seeds

- 2 tablespoons cashew nuts

Directions:

• Press the Sauté button and heat the olive oil. Once the oil is hot, sear the tofu on all edges until lightly golden. This takes about 5 minutes.

• Once the tofu is golden, sauté the garlic and ginger until fragrant.

• Add the broccoli and corn. Season with soy sauce and black pepper. Pour in enough water.

• Close the lid and set the vent to the Sealing position.

• Press the Pressure Cook or Manual button and adjust the cooking time to 6 minutes.

• Do quick pressure release.

• Once the lid is open, press the Sauté button and stir in the cornstarch slurry. Simmer for 3 minutes until the sauce thickens.

• Sprinkle with sesame seeds and cashew nuts before serving;

Nutrition:

Calories 296 | Total Fat 24g | Saturated Fat 4g | Total Carbs 8g | Net Carbs 5g | Protein 16g | Sugar: 2g | Fiber: 3g | Sodium: 138mg | Potassium: 278mg | Phosphorus: 231mg

Green Dream Noodles

Preparation Time: 5 minutes | Cooking Time: 25 minutes | Servings: 4

Ingredients:

- 1 tablespoon olive oil

- 3 cloves garlic, minced

- 1 1-inch ginger, sliced thinly

- ½ cup sliced mushrooms

- 1 sachet miso paste

- 1 ½ cups vegetable broth

- 1 cup broccoli florets

- 1 handful sugar snap peas

- 2 cup of rice noodles

- A handful of fresh coriander leaves

Directions:

• Press the Sauté button on the Pressure pot and heat the oil. Sauté the garlic and ginger for a minute or until fragrant.

• Stir in the mushrooms and add the miso paste and vegetable broth.

• Simmer for 3 minutes.

• Stir in the broccoli florets, peas, and noodles.

• Close the lid and set the vent to the Sealing position.

• Press the Soup/Broth button and cook for 20 minutes.

• Do natural pressure release.

• Garnish with coriander leaves before serving.

Nutrition:

Calories 131 | Total Fat 4g | Saturated Fat 0.5g | Total Carbs 22g | Net Carbs 21g | Protein 2g | Sugar: 0.1g | Fiber: 1g | Sodium: 21mg | Potassium: 39mg | Phosphorus: 30mg

Slow Cook Glazed Carrots and Parsnips

Preparation Time: 5 minutes | Cooking Time: 5 hours | Servings: 4

Ingredients:

- 2 large carrots, peeled and cut into thick strips

- 1 large parsnip, peeled and cut into thick strips

- ¼ cup maple syrup

- salt and pepper to taste

Directions:

- Place all ingredients in the Pressure pot and give a good stir.

- Close the lid but do not seal the vent.

- Press the Slow Cook button and adjust the cooking time to 5 hours.

- Halfway through the cooking time, stir the vegetables.

Nutrition:

Calories 102 | Total Fat 0.2g | Saturated Fat 0g | Total Carbs 25g | Net Carbs 22g | Protein 0.8g | Sugar: 15g | Fiber: 3g | Sodium: 10mg | Potassium: 298mg | Phosphorus: 48mg

Sweet Potato, Squash, Coconut, And Cardamom

Preparation Time: 10 minutes | Cooking Time: 12 minutes | Servings: 4

Ingredients:

- 2 tablespoons coconut oil

- 3 cloves garlic, minced

- 1 onion, chopped

- 1 1-inch thick ginger

- 3 cardamom pods

- 1 cup diced sweet potatoes

- 1 cup diced kabocha squash

- 1 14-ounce coconut milk

- salt and pepper to taste

Directions:

• Press the Sauté button on the Pressure pot. Heat the oil and sauté the garlic and onion for 1 minute or until translucent.

• Add the ginger and cardamom pods until fragrant.

• Stir in the rest of the ingredients.

• Close the lid and set the vent to the Sealing position.

• Press the Pressure Cook or Manual button and adjust the cooking time to 10 minutes.

• Do natural pressure release.

Nutrition:

Calories 102 | Total Fat 7g | Saturated Fat 6g | Total Carbs 9g | Net Carbs 6g | Protein 2g | Sugar: 4g | Fiber: 3g | Sodium: 109mg | Potassium: 392mg | Phosphorus: 49mg

Jersey Royals with Wild Garlic

Preparation Time: 5 minutes | Cooking Time: 5 hours | Servings: 2

Ingredients:

• 5 tablespoons olive oil

• ½ pound Jersey royal potatoes scrubbed clean and cut into wedges

• A handful of garlic leaves

• A few sprigs of rosemary

• salt and pepper to taste

Directions:

• Place all ingredients in the Pressure pot. Stir to combine everything.

• Close the lid but do not seal the vent.

• Press the Slow Cook button and adjust the cooking time to 5 hours.

• Stir the potatoes halfway through the cooking time.

Nutrition:

Calories 386 | Total Fat 34g | Saturated Fat 5g | Total Carbs 20g | Net Carbs 17g | Protein 2g | Sugar: 0.8g | Fiber: 3g | Sodium: 7mg | Potassium: 478mg | Phosphorus: 65mg

Miso-Glazed Eggplants

Preparation Time: 5 minutes | Cooking Time: 5 minutes | Servings: 2

Ingredients:

• 4 medium eggplants, sliced into 1-inch pieces

• 2 cloves garlic, minced

• 1 teaspoon miso paste

• 1 teaspoon brown sugar

• 1 teaspoon soy sauce

• 1 teaspoon sesame oil

• Salt and pepper to taste

• 1 teaspoon toasted sesame seed

Directions:

• Place all ingredients except for the toasted sesame seeds in the Pressure pot and give a good stir.

• Close the lid and set the vent to the Sealing position.

• Press the Pressure Cook or Manual button. Adjust the cooking time to 5 minutes.

• Do natural pressure release.

• Garnish with sesame seeds before serving.

Nutrition:

Calories 324 | Total Fat 6g | Saturated Fat 1g | Total Carbs 68g | Net Carbs 35g | Protein 12g | Sugar: 41g | Fiber: 33g | Sodium: 117mg | Potassium: 2540mg | Phosphorus: 286mg

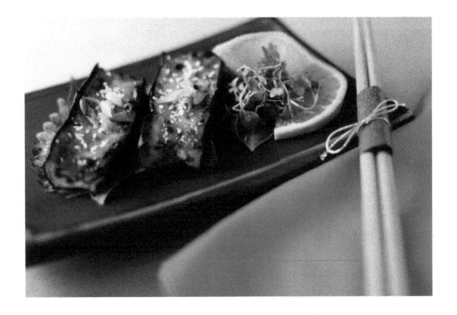

Butternut Squash and Thyme

Preparation Time: 5 minutes | Cooking Time: 6 minutes | Servings: 4

Ingredients:

- 2 tablespoons olive oil

- 2 cloves of garlic, minced

- 1 sprig of thyme

- ½ medium butternut squash, peeled and sliced

- ½ cup vegetable broth

- salt and pepper to taste

Directions:

- Press the Sauté button on the Pressure pot and heat the oil.

- Sauté the garlic for 30 seconds until fragrant.

- Stir in the rest of the ingredients.

- Close the lid and set the vent to the Sealing position.

• Press the Pressure Cook or Manual button and cook on high for 5 minutes.

• Do natural pressure release.

Nutrition:

Calories 120 | Total Fat 7g | Saturated Fat 1g | Total Carbs 15g | Net Carbs 12g | Protein 1g | Sugar: 3g | Fiber: 3g | Sodium: 74mg | Potassium: 446mg | Phosphorus: 44mg

Lemony Artichokes with Olives Pasta

Preparation Time: 10 minutes | Cooking Time: 12 minutes | Servings: 4

Ingredients:

• 6 ounces linguine pasta

• 4 cups of water

• 2 tablespoon olive oil

• 1 onion, minced

• 2 cloves garlic, minced

• 1 14-ounce can artichoke hearts, drained and halved

• Salt and pepper to taste

• 1 tablespoon grated lemon zest

• 3 tablespoons lemon juice

• ½ cup green olives, pitted and chopped

• 1 teaspoon red pepper flakes

• 2 tablespoon parsley, chopped

Directions:

• Place the pasta and water in the Pressure pot.

• Close the lid and set the vent to the Sealing position. Press the Pressure Cook or Manual button and adjust the cooking time to 6 minutes. Do quick pressure release. Once the lid is open, drain the pasta then set it aside. Clean the inner pot.

• Press the Sauté button on the Instant and heat olive oil.

• Sauté the onion and garlic for a minute or until lightly golden.

• Stir in the artichokes and season with salt and pepper to taste. Stir for 3 minutes.

• Add in the rest of the ingredients.

• Stir for 3 minutes or until everything is combined.

Nutrition:

Calories 184 | Total Fat 8g | Saturated Fat 1g | Total Carbs 28g | Net Carbs 17g | Protein 5g | Sugar: 3g | Fiber: 11g | Sodium: 68mg | Potassium: 371mg | Phosphorus: 118mg

One-Pot Curried Butternut Squash

Preparation Time: 5 minutes | Cooking Time: 5 minutes | Servings: 4

Ingredients:

- 1 14-ounce coconut milk

- 1 1-inch ginger, sliced

- 1 onion, minced

- 2 cloves garlic, minced

- ½ butternut squash, peeled and sliced

- 1 tablespoon turmeric powder

- 1 tablespoon garam masala powder

- 2 tablespoons lemon juice

- salt and pepper to taste

Directions:

- Place all ingredients in the Pressure pot. Give a good stir.

- Close the lid and set the vent to the Sealing position.

- Press the Pressure Cook or Manual button.

- Adjust the cooking time to 5 minutes.

- Once the timer sets off, do natural pressure release.

Nutrition:

Calories 42 | Total Fat 0.3g | Saturated Fat 0g | Total Carbs 9g | Net Carbs 7g | Protein 1g | Sugar: 4g | Fiber: 2g | Sodium: 106mg | Potassium: 354mg | Phosphorus: 38mg

Steamed Eggplant Salad

Preparation Time: minutes | Cooking Time: minutes | Servings: 2

Ingredients:

• 1 cup of water

• 4 medium-sized Chinese eggplants

• ½ cup chopped tomatoes

• 1 red onion, chopped

• 1 tablespoon grated ginger

• Juice from ½ lemon, freshly squeezed

• 1 tablespoon chopped green onions

• salt and pepper to taste

Directions:

• Pour water into the Pressure pot and place a steamer basket or trivet inside.

• Place the Chinese eggplants on the basket.

• Close the lid and set the vent to the Sealing position.

• Press the Steam button. Cook for 10 minutes.

• Do natural pressure release.

• Once the lid is open, take the eggplants out and allow them to cool.

• Once cool, shred with two forks. Place in a bowl and add the rest of the ingredients.

Nutrition:

Calories 309 | Total Fat 2g | Saturated Fat 0.5g | Total Carbs 73g | Net Carbs 39g | Protein 12g | Sugar: 42g | Fiber: 34g | Sodium: 27mg | Potassium: 2708mg | Phosphorus: 291mg

Plain Spaghetti Squash

Preparation Time: 5 minutes | Cooking Time: 10 minutes | Servings: 2

Ingredients:

- 1 cup of water

- 1 spaghetti squash, cut lengthwise and seeds removed

- Salt and pepper to taste

Directions:

- Pour water into the Pressure pot and place a steamer basket or trivet inside.

- Season the spaghetti squash with salt and pepper.

- Place on the steamer basket.

- Close the lid and set the vent to the Sealing position.

- Press the Steam button cook for 10 minutes.

- Do natural pressure release.

- Once the lid is open, remove the squash and fluff using a fork.

Nutrition:

Calories 9 | Total Fat 0.05g | Saturated Fat 0g | Total Carbs 2g | Net Carbs 1.7g | Protein 0.5g | Sugar: 1g | Fiber: 0.3g | Sodium: 4mg | Potassium: 77mg | Phosphorus: 10mg

Korean Braised Potatoes

Preparation Time: 5 minutes | Cooking Time: 30 minutes | Servings: 4

Ingredients:

• pound baby potatoes scrubbed clean

• 3 tablespoons soy sauce

• 2 tablespoons sugar

• 3 cloves garlic, minced

• 1 cup of water

• Sesame seeds for garnish

Directions:

• Place all ingredients except for the sesame seeds in the Pressure pot.

• Close the lid and set the vent to the Sealing position.

• Press the Meat/Stew button and adjust the time to 20 minutes.

• Once the timer sets off, do a quick pressure release to open the lid.

• Once the lid is open, press the Sauté button and allow the sauce to simmer until it has

reduced to a glaze. Stir constantly.

• Garnish with sesame seeds before serving.

Nutrition:

Calories 141 | Total Fat 2g | Saturated Fat 0.4g | Total Carbs 28g | Net Carbs 25g | Protein 3g | Sugar: 7g | Fiber: 3g | Sodium: 188mg | Potassium: 518mg | Phosphorus: 83mg

Broccoli and Rice

Preparation Time: 5 minutes | Cooking Time: 8 minutes | Servings: 6

Ingredients:

- 1 teaspoon coconut oil

- 2 cloves garlic, minced

- 3 cups broccoli florets

- 8 ounces shiitake mushrooms

- 10 ounces pre-cooked or leftover rice

- 1 cup roasted cashews

- 3 tablespoons soy sauce

- pepper to taste

- 3 tablespoons toasted sesame oil

Directions:

- Press the Sauté button on the Pressure pot and heat the coconut oil.

• Stir in the garlic and sauté for 30 seconds until fragrant.

• Add in the broccoli and shiitake mushrooms. Cook for 3 minutes until the broccoli has

wilted.

• Add in the leftover rice and cashew and season with soy sauce and pepper to taste.

• Stir for 3 minutes.

• Drizzle with sesame oil before serving.

Nutrition:

Calories 428 | Total Fat 32g | Saturated Fat 6g | Total Carbs 33g | Net Carbs 30g | Protein 8g | Sugar: 7g | Fiber: 3g | Sodium: 264mg | Potassium: 301mg | Phosphorus: 212mg

Vegetable Paella

Preparation Time: 10 minutes | Cooking Time: 35 minutes | Servings: 6

Ingredients:

- 3 tablespoons olive oil

- 1 onion, chopped finely

- 6 cloves garlic, minced

- 2 teaspoons smoked paprika

- 1 15-ounces diced tomatoes

- 2 cups short-grain rice

- 1 can chickpeas

- 3 cups vegetable broth

- ½ cup dry white wine

- ½ teaspoon saffron threads

- salt and pepper to taste

- 1 14-ounce artichoke, drained

- ½ cup Kalamata olives pitted and halved

- ½ cup frozen peas

- 2 red bell peppers, seeded and cut into strips

- 2 tablespoons lemon juice

- ¼ cup fresh parsley, chopped

Directions:

- Press the Sauté button on the Pressure pot and heat the oil. Sauté the onion and garlic until fragrant. Stir in the paprika, tomatoes, rice, and chickpeas. Stir for 2 minutes. Add in the broth, white wine, and saffron. Stir to combine or until the liquid is simmering. Season with salt and pepper to taste.

- Arrange the artichokes, olives, peas, and bell pepper on top. Drizzle with lemon juice.

- Close the lid and set the vent to the Sealing position.

- Press the Rice button and cook on low until the timer sets off.

- Do natural pressure release.

- Garnish with parsley before serving.

Nutrition:

Calories 546 | Total Fat 13g | Saturated Fat 3g | Total Carbs 93g | Net Carbs 81g | Protein 18g | Sugar: 8g | Fiber: 12g | Sodium: 339mg | Potassium: 908mg | Phosphorus: 306mg

Cauliflower in Cashew Chipotle Sauce

Preparation Time: 5 minutes | Cooking Time: 6 minutes | Servings: 4

Ingredients:

- 1 cup cashew nut, soaked overnight and drained

- 3 tablespoons nutritional yeast

- 2 tablespoons lime juice

- 3 tablespoons adobo or chipotle hot sauce

- 2 tablespoons olive oil

- salt and pepper to taste

- 1 large head cauliflower, cut into florets

- 1 cup of water

Directions:

• In a blender, place the cashew nuts, water, nutritional yeast, lime juice, adobo or chipotle sauce, and olive oil. Season with salt and pepper to taste. Pulse until smooth. Set aside.

• Place the cauliflower and water in the Pressure pot and pour over the cashew chipotle sauce.

• Close the lid and set the vent to the Sealing position.

• Press the Pressure Cook or Manual button and adjust the cooking time to 6 minutes.

• Once the timer sets off, do a quick pressure release.

Nutrition:

Calories 294 | Total Fat 22g | Saturated Fat 4g | Total Carbs 17g | Net Carbs 13g | Protein 10g | Sugar: 4g | Fiber: 4g | Sodium: 615mg | Potassium: 733mg | Phosphorus: 220mg

Slow-Cooked Veggie Enchilada Casserole

Preparation Time: 5 minutes | Cooking Time: 5 hours | Servings: 5

Ingredients:

- ½ medium head of cauliflower, cut into florets

- 1 large sweet potato, peeled and cubed

- 2 red bell peppers, cut into squares

- 3 tablespoons extra virgin olive oil

- 1 teaspoon ground cumin

- 8 ounces red salsa

- salt and pepper to taste

- 2 handful baby spinach leaves

- ½ cup fresh cilantro

- 9 corn tortillas, halved

Directions:

• Place the cauliflower, sweet potato, bell peppers, olive oil, cumin, and salsa in the Instant

Pot. Season with salt and pepper to taste. Add in the baby spinach on top.

• Close the lid but do not seal the vent.

• Press the Slow Cook function and adjust the cooking time to 5 hours.

• Once cooked, serve with cilantro and tortillas.

Nutrition:

Calories 94 | Total Fat 4g | Saturated Fat 0.5g | Total Carbs 14g | Net Carbs 11g | Protein 2g | Sugar: 6g | Fiber: 3g | Sodium: 416mg | Potassium: 456mg | Phosphorus: 58mg

Bok Choy With Mushrooms

Preparation Time: 5 minutes | Cooking Time: 10 minutes | Servings: 4

Ingredients:

- 3 tablespoons olive oil

- 1 small yellow onion, chopped

- 2 cloves garlic, minced

- 5 ounces fresh shiitake mushrooms

- 1 red bell pepper, seeded and sliced into strips

- pound bok choy, torn

- 1 cup vegetable broth

- 2 tablespoons soy sauce

- salt and pepper to taste

- 1 tablespoon sesame seed oil

- 1 tablespoon cornstarch + 2 tablespoons water

Directions:

• Press the Sauté button on the Pressure pot. Heat the oil and sauté the onion and garlic for 30 seconds or until fragrant.

• Stir in the mushrooms and red bell pepper. Sauté for 3 minutes.

• Add in the bok choy and vegetable broth. Season with soy sauce, salt, and pepper to taste.

• Close the lid and set the vent to the Sealing position.

• Press the Pressure Cook or Manual button and adjust the cooking time to 3 minutes.

• Do quick pressure release.

• Once the lid is open, press the Sauté button and stir in the sesame oil and cornstarch slurry. Stir for 3 minutes until the sauce thickens.

Nutrition:

Calories 138 | Total Fat 11g | Saturated Fat 2g | Total Carbs 10g | Net Carbs 8g | Protein 3g | Sugar: 4g | Fiber: 2g | Sodium: 131mg | Potassium: 447mg | Phosphorus: 63mg

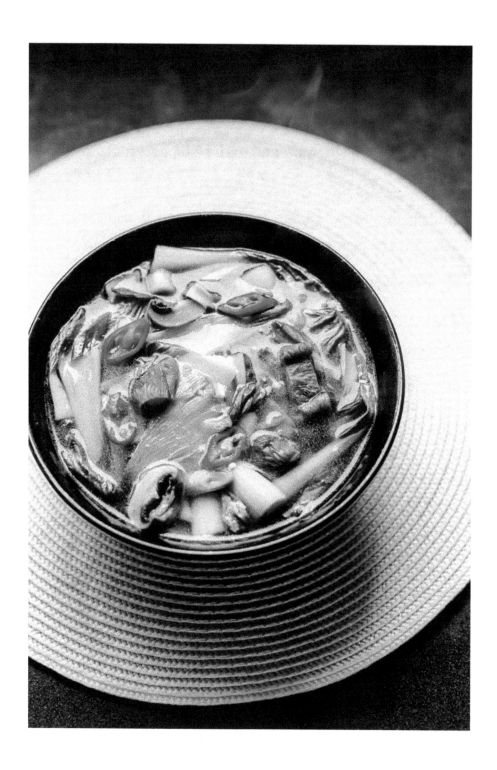